Therapeutic Horseback Riding

A Comprehensive Guide for Individuals, Instructors, and Facilities

Table of Contents

Chapter 1. Introduction

Welcome to our special report on "Therapeutic Horseback Riding: A Comprehensive Guide for Individuals, Instructors, and Facilities"! This enlightening guide is far more than merely saddle talks and horse whispers. It's a captivating journey into an intriguing world where the majestic stride of a horse meets the resilience of the human spirit. From therapists and caregivers seeking a novel approach to uplift their beneficiaries' lives, to equestrian centers aspiring to expand their scope, our report leaves no stone unturned. After relishing this cheerful harmonization of human and equine wellbeing, you'll be enticed into experiencing the transformative power of therapeutic horseback riding yourself or implementing it within your facility. Purchase your copy today and let's gallop together into a new horizon of healing and growth!

Chapter 2. Understanding the Basics of Therapeutic Horseback Riding

Before delving into the various aspects surrounding therapeutic horseback riding (THR), it's crucial to understand the basics that define this practice. This includes, but is not limited to, an overview of what THR entails, the science behind its effectiveness, the roles of various personnel, and some key considerations from a safety perspective.

2.1. What is Therapeutic Horseback Riding?

Therapeutic Horseback Riding, known also by the term Equine-Assisted Therapy (EAT), comprises interventions that involve equine activities designed and directed by professionals with the intention of improving the individual participant's physical, emotional, social, cognitive, and behavioral health.

Horses provide a unique rhythmic, multidimensional movement pattern similar to the natural walk of a human, thus helping participants to develop balance, coordination, strength, and self-confidence. The experience is not limited to mere physical gains; THR activities can be instrumental in improving emotional well-being and cognitive abilities too.

2.2. The Science Behind Therapeutic Horseback Riding

The premise of THR lies in the unique movement provided by the horse, which cannot be reproduced mechanically. When riding, the horse's gait helps to stimulate a rider's pelvis and trunk in a manner reminiscent of a human walking. This physical engagement strengthens core muscles, improves postural control, balance, and overall motor function.

On the psychological front, the experience of interacting with a horse can instill a sense of responsibility, empathy, and self-efficacy in the rider. The interplay of these elements often leads to reduced anxiety, better emotional management, and improved social skills.

Cognitively, horseback riding and related activities can enhance problem-solving, planning, and adaptability by challenging riders to make decisions, follow routines, and adapt to the horse's responses.

2.3. Key Roles in Therapeutic Horseback Riding

A successful THR program involves many individuals each playing a vital role. Understanding these roles can shed light on the intricacies involved in delivering effective therapy sessions:

1. Therapist/Instructor: The therapist is a certified professional who designs and conducts the THR program. They ensure the safety and efficacy of sessions, guided by an understanding of the rider's needs.

2. Horse: The horse plays the most direct role in therapy. Not just any horse can be used for THR. The selected horses undergo rigorous training and are chosen based on disposition, tolerance, gait, and size.

3. Volunteers: Volunteers are essential in maintaining safety during sessions, helping with horse care, and assisting with special events in the program.

4. Riders: Participants can range widely in age and abilities, each

with unique therapeutic goals. They are active members of the therapy process, growing and healing through their interactions.

5. Caretakers: These family members or paid caregivers are fundamental to provide care and support to the participants. They communicate with the Therapist about any changes or concerns and assist in implementing therapeutic strategies at home.

2.4. Safety Considerations

Safety is paramount when dealing with an activity that involves large animals and individuals who may have special needs. A safe environment sets the foundation for an effective therapeutic experience, facilitating progress toward therapeutic goals.

It involves:

1. Staff Training: All involved in the program must be adequately trained in horse handling, emergency procedures, rider support, and any specialized needs of the riders.

2. Appropriate Equipment: Use of safety gear such as helmets, carefully selected saddles and adaptations for individual riders' needs are essential to maintaining physical safety.

3. Matching Horses and Riders: Factors like the horse's abilities, temperament, size, and the individual rider's needs and goals should guide the selection process.

4. Maintaining Horse Health: Besides regular veterinary care, the horses' workload, rest, nutrition, and overall well-being need to be well managed to ensure they remain fit and healthy for therapy.

With a clear understanding of what goes into therapeutic horseback riding and a firm grip on these basics, it's possible to delve deeper into the subject and truly appreciate the power of THR in enhancing health, wellness, and the quality of life.

Chapter 3. The History and Evolution of Equine Therapy

The genesis of equine therapy has its roots in the antiquity, gaining more prominence in the modern era due to the reported benefits of human-equine interaction. This age-old practice, though varied, has consistently demonstrated that it is not merely a complementary segment of treatment, but an effective standalone therapeutic strategy as well.

3.1. Ancient Roots

Dating back to ancient times, people quickly recognized the profound psychological and physiological effects horses could have on humans. Ancient Greeks used horses, considered a divine symbol of power and nobility, to uplift the spirits of the differently-abled and those afflicted by disease. Hippocrates, the Greek "father of medicine", wrote about the rhythmic movement of riding, proclaiming it as a form of therapeutic exercise. This recognition morphed into what is known today as Hippotherapy, a term deduced from the Greek word 'hippo' for horse.

3.2. Middle Ages to Modern Era

During the Middle Ages and the Renaissance, horses continued to play a therapeutic role in enhancing physical strength and improving morale, especially for knights and warriors during periods of convalescence. However, it was in the mid-1800s that the formalization of equine therapy began to gain ground. It was acknowledged within the German and French medical literature detailing how horseback riding was instrumental in improving posture, balance, and joint flexibility.

In more recent history, as the horrors of World War I and II unfolded, the military forces observed an incidental improvement in the emotional state and morale of wounded soldiers when they interacted with horses. This sparked deeper interest, leading to the pairing of therapeutic riding with traditional forms of therapy, creating a holistic path of rehabilitation.

3.3. Therapeutic Riding Schools

Following World War II, therapeutic riding began taking a more structured form across Europe. Liz Hartel, a Danish woman afflicted with polio, despite her paralysis, won the silver medal in dressage in the 1952 Helsinki Olympics. This incredible achievement kicked off a wave of therapeutic riding schools. The global recognition of her incorrigible spirit and supreme equine skills led to the establishment of the first therapeutic riding center in Denmark by Hartel and her therapist, Dr. Eigil Nielsen.

The 1960s marked the birth of therapeutic riding in North America. Canadian-born physical therapist Lis Hartel and occupational therapist Eileen Watkin launched one of the earliest therapeutic riding centers in North America at Sunnybrook Medical Centre in Toronto, Canada.

The US followed in the footsteps of Canada, with the Cheff Therapeutic Riding Center in Michigan staking its claim as the first center in the country solely dedicated to equine therapy.

3.4. Professionalization of the Field

The 1980s and 1990s oversaw the formalization of the therapeutic riding industry worldwide. Major organizations, such as the North American Riding for the Handicapped Association (NARHA), the British Horse Society (BHS), and the Federation of Horses in Education and Therapy International (HETI), evolved to provide guidelines, training, and certification for instructors.

In 1990, the American Hippotherapy Association was formed to promote the use of horses as viable therapeutic tools for medical professionals

Over time, these institutions have greatly influenced the standards and best practices that have shaped therapeutic riding into what it is today.

3.5. Expansion of the Field

Equine-assisted therapy has matured beyond mere horseback riding. Adjacent fields, such as Equine Facilitated Psychotherapy (EFP) and Equine Assisted Learning (EAL), have blossomed over the years.

EFP facilitates psychological healing by utilizing horses in the therapeutic process, often dealing with emotional and behavioral challenges. On the other hand, EAL employs horses to assist in learning or education, accommodating a wide range of individuals, from corporate teams aiming for better group dynamics to 'at-risk' youth working on behavioral improvements.

3.6. Towards A Bright Future

Today, equine-assisted therapy persists as an exponentially growing field, extending its healing touch to individuals across different demographics and therapeutic needs. Technology is making equine therapy more accessible, with tools like equine simulators providing individuals with an immersive equestrian experience, particularly beneficial for those unable to engage directly with live horses.

The history and evolution of equine therapy, while rooted in ancient practices, remains an ever-evolving field. As we look forward, the potentials for expansion seem boundless. With the continual integration of technology, advancements in scientific understanding, and innovative therapeutic techniques, the sky's indeed the limit for this remarkable intersection of the equine spirit and human resilience. After all, as Winston Churchill very aptly remarked, "There is something about the outside of a horse that is good for the inside of a man."

Chapter 4. Selecting the Right Horse: Temperament and Traits

An integral component in therapeutic horseback riding is selecting the right horse. Not every horse is suited for the work involved in this form of therapy, and the choice should be made with careful consideration and expert guidance. This chapter serves as a practical guide for understanding and evaluating the different horse temperaments and traits necessary for success in a therapeutic riding program.

4.1. Assessment of Horse's Temperament

The temperament of a horse plays a pivotal role in therapeutic riding. It's not just a horse's physical ability that matters for this kind of work; their mental state is equally important. A horse used in therapeutic riding should exhibit calmness, patience, and confidence in their demeanor. In order to assess a horse's temperament, take note of these key factors:

- Patience: A therapeutic horse needs to have a high level of patience as they interact with riders with diverse abilities and special needs. Riders may make unpredictable movements or take longer to mount and dismount.

- Curiosity: A horse's natural inquisitive nature can be an asset in therapy sessions. This characteristic often indicates a higher ability to adapt to new situations.

- Confidence: Therapeutic horses need to demonstrate a stable and reliable behavior at all times. They should not be easily startled or skittish.

- Tolerance: A horse for therapeutic riding should tolerate various noises, movements, objects, or uneven weight distribution without becoming disturbed or agitated.

4.2. Horse Personality Types

The psychology of horses is complex, but studies have defined three broad horse personality types: hot-blooded, cold-blooded, and warm-blooded. Knowing these categories can significantly assist while selecting the right candidate for therapeutic riding.

- Hot-Blooded Horses: These are often racehorses, like Arabians and Thoroughbreds. They are known for their speed, energy, and agility, but also for their sensitivity and reactive nature, which may not be suitable for therapeutic riding.

- Cold-Blooded Horses: Usually representing draft breeds, cold-blooded horses are calm and patient. Their slow, steady movements make them an apt choice for many therapeutic programs.

- Warm-Blooded Horses: These are a mix of hot and cold breeds, demonstrating aspects of both personality types. Warm-blooded horses have the calm demeanor of a cold-blooded horse but with the agility of a hot-blooded one.

4.3. Factors to Evaluate Horse Traits

Choosing the right horse for therapeutic riding significantly hinges on evaluating the horse traits considering the following factors:

- Age: Younger horses may lack the maturity and patience needed for this work. Older horses, with more life experience, are usually calmer and more adaptable.

- Size: The size of the horse should be suitable for the riders. Bigger horses may intimidate some riders or be difficult for them to mount and dismount.

- Training: A horse's training history is critical. Look for a horse trained in a gentle and friendly environment, signalling its adaptability to therapeutic sessions.

- Health History: Knowing about a horse's past and current health conditions is vital. A horse that is in pain or uncomfortable can potentially cause instability during the therapy sessions.

4.4. Experience and Observation

While the aforementioned factors lay the foundation, it is the long-term interaction with the horse, including consistent observations and encounters that will provide you a more accurate picture of whether the horse is suitable for therapeutic horseback riding or not.

Always start with a trial period for any new horse so that the horse, therapists, and riders get adequate time to know each other. Monitor the horse's behavior during varied situations and note changes, if any.

4.5. Final Notes

Remember, each horse is unique. Horses, like humans, have their unique personalities and quirks so be patient during the selection process. The secret to a successful therapeutic riding program is not only finding the "right" horse but also developing a strong rapport between the horse, rider, and the therapeutic staff.

Acquiring a good match will take time and thoughtful evaluation, but the rewards that therapeutic horseback riding brings is indeed well worth it. This chapter has equipped you with all the tools you need to make a well-informed choice, taking you one step closer to uniting the perfect horse and rider, and maximizing the therapeutic journey. End your selection process not when you find the right horse, rather when you can't imagine the journey ahead without them.

Chapter 5. The Role of Riding Instructors and Therapists: Bridging the Gap

Traditional therapeutic practices have witnessed a paradigm shift in recent years with the inclusion of various unique forms of therapy, one of them being therapeutic horseback riding. As an intersection between the world of healthcare and equestrian sports, many different personalities play their roles. Among them, two vital characters who ensure the seamless operation of this therapy are the riding instructors and therapists. While both have distinct roles, working together creates a bridge towards better healing and growth of their clients.

5.1. The Role of the Riding Instructor

The role of the riding instructor extends beyond merely teaching horseback riding skills. They ensure participants are comfortable and well-equipped to connect with the horse. They are trained not just in horse handling but also psychology and individual learning variations among participants. This supports them to fortify the bond between the participant and the horse. Safety, undoubtedly, rests as their paramount concern, making sure their students are secure in all stages, from saddling and warming up to the cooling-down phase beyond the course.

The skill-set of a good riding instructor includes:

- Knowledge about horses and horse behavior
- Understanding the physical abilities and psychological needs of participants

- Teaching and communication skills
- Patience and empathy

5.2. The Role of the Therapist

The role of the therapist within therapeutic horseback riding is manifold. Generally, they examine the participant's mental and emotional state, identifying their areas of struggle. They use the therapeutic horse riding session to work on these issues, with the help of the instructor.

The therapist is fundamentally trained in a healthcare sphere, like psychotherapy, occupational therapy, or physical therapy. They also need to be familiar with equine behavior and the benefits of therapeutic horseback riding, to mold and implement the therapy.

The skill-set of a good therapist includes:

- Therapeutic skills specific to their area of specialization
- Understanding the dynamics of the horse-human connection
- Communication and coordination skills
- Empathy, patience, and the ability to encourage participants

5.3. Working Together: Bridging the Gap

The tandem of the instructor and therapist is crucial in therapeutic horseback riding. The instructor provides the ground with his or her technical know-how of horse-riding, and the therapist extends his or her expertise by using the dynamic horse-human interaction therapeutically. They must work in tandem, aiding and enhancing each other's work.

The alliance is rooted in constant communication. Both parties should understand what the participant's objectives are, both physically and emotionally. Aided by regular meetings, the therapist and the riding instructor can outline a personalized program for each individual.

5.4. The Participant's Perspective

From the participant's perspective, the partnership between the riding instructor and the therapist should be seamless. They have to view their riding instructor not just as a mentor in horseback riding, but also as an integral part of their therapeutic journey. Similarly, they have to see the therapist not just as a healthcare professional, but as someone who understands their bond with the horse.

5.5. Barriers and Solutions

Naturally, barriers can creep in with two different disciplines working together. Lack of mutual understanding, communication gaps, differences over therapy protocols are some challenges that may hinder a smooth partnership.

Having regular joint schedules, shared therapy plans, and understanding of each other's specialties, and efficient communication are ways to overcome these barriers.

5.6. Continued Learning and Growth

Instructor and therapist learning does not stop at certain, predefined thresholds. As new studies emerge and techniques evolve, both should strive for continued education. By attending workshops, conferences, and various training programs, they can broaden their skills and thus, ensure better service.

In conclusion, the symbiotic relationship of riding instructors and therapists serves as the bedrock of therapeutic horseback riding. An ideal bridge between these two roles is formed by mutual understanding, continuous communication, respect for each other's specialities, and a shared goal of the participant's wellbeing. Through collaborative efforts, they facilitate a rich, empowering environment where individuals can grow physically, emotionally, and socially.

Chapter 6. The Physical and Mental Benefits of Therapeutic Riding

Therapeutic riding is a unique form of therapy that has been leveraged for centuries to help individuals of all ages deal with a variety of physical, mental, and emotional challenges. It is a multifaceted approach to healing that fosters a connection between the human participant and the horse, eliciting benefits that transcend the traditional settings of therapy.

6.1. The Physical Benefits of Therapeutic Riding

The physical benefits of therapeutic riding are extensive and multifarious, cutting across various realms of human health and wellness. These benefits are often measurable and can result in substantial improvements in physical health and capability.

One of the single most obvious benefits relates to the promotion of balance. Riding a horse requires maintenance of a stable core. The rhythmic, symmetrical movement of the horse provides an external stimulus to stimulate and improve both static and dynamic balance. It's an engaging workout, stirring muscles you wouldn't activate in regular physical therapy.

Walking a horse leads to improved gait patterns due to the horse's movement mimicking the human walk. Riders subconsciously adjust their pelvic movements to correspond with the horse's stride, leading to enhanced motor planning and increased strength in trunk and postural muscles. This can be extremely beneficial for people with disabilities affecting their mobility, such as cerebral palsy or multiple sclerosis.

The coordination necessary to ride can also significantly improve fine and gross motor skills. Horse riding requires a combination of movements and cognitive processes that demand communication and synchronization of different body parts, helping to improve hand-eye coordination, lateralization and body awareness.

Added to these benefits is the aspect of improved muscle tone and strength. Horseback riding and care of horses invoke all core muscle groups and help gain muscle strength without overtaxing the cardiovascular system.

6.2. The Mental Benefits of Therapeutic Riding

While the physical benefits are tangible and apparent, the mental and psychological benefits of therapeutic riding cannot be overstated. Partaking in these equine activities serves as an excellent form of psychotherapy. The bond formed between the rider and the horse often acts as a medium for emotional healing.

Serving as a strong motivator, horse riding can boost self-esteem and self-image. There's a certain sense of achievement in controlling and navigating such a large and formidable creature, helping to instill a sense of empowerment, independence, and an improved sense of self-worth.

The act of horseback riding can be incredibly relaxing, which in turn reduces stress levels. The rhythmic motion and the direct contact with another living being promote a state of mindfulness that can help people manage feelings of anxiety, depression, and stress.

Memory, concentration, and learning abilities are also enhanced along the way. The need to remember riding patterns, commands, and techniques creates a mentally stimulating environment, promoting cognitive agility. People with cognitive disorders or learning disabilities can benefit from improved attention span, problem-solving capabilities, and flexible thinking.

An often unmentioned benefit includes the development of social skills. Although therapeutic riding may seem to be a solitary activity, it includes interactions with instructors, therapists, and other riders, which all work towards enhancing the rider's ability to communicate and integrate within a social setting.

All in all, therapeutic horseback riding fosters resilience and engenders a sense of joy and contentment.

6.3. The Synergy of Physical and Mental Benefits

The physical and mental benefits of therapeutic riding intertwine to bring about an overall improvement in the quality of life. Physical advancements like improved balance and muscle strength often lead to increased independence and self-sufficiency, which in turn add to the rider's confidence and self-esteem.

Similarly, the mental benefits such as stress reduction can reflect in better physical health, with stress being a contributor to a host of physical health issues. Therefore, improvements in one area can often lead to progress in another, underlying the interconnectivity between physical and mental health.

From enhancing body functions to uplifting mental wellbeing, therapeutic horseback riding provides myriad benefits. It blurs the line between therapeutic treatment and an enriching life experience, making it a uniquely holistic intervention in the grand spectrum of healing therapies.

Chapter 7. Setting up a Therapeutic Riding Program: Best Practices

Establishing a therapeutic riding program requires comprehensive planning and preparation. Key considerations should include safety procedures, rider assessment, session planning, horse selection and training, volunteer management, and facility requirements. Each aspect must be carefully managed to ensure the delivery of beneficial interventions while maintaining a safe, adaptive, and comforting environment for all participants.

7.1. Safety Procedures

Safety should always be a priority in a therapeutic riding program. Regular safety inspections of equipment and horses, as well as training of all personnel in emergency procedures, are vital. Moreover, instructors should be certified by recognized organizations, such as the Professional Association of Therapeutic Horsemanship International (PATH Intl.). The guidelines set by these organizations can help maintain the highest safety and ethical standards.

7.2. Rider Assessment

Before starting the riding sessions, potential riders should undergo a comprehensive evaluation. This assessment usually includes medical history, physical capacity, psychological profile, and personal goals. It's crucial to involve health professionals in this process to assure riders can safely participate and benefit from the program.

7.3. Session Planning

After the initial assessment, it's time to create personalized therapeutic plans. These plans should focus not only on riding skills but on the specific therapeutic outcomes desired. For instance, if a rider needs to improve balance and coordination, the session's activities should be designed around this goal. Remember that progress may be slow, so it's important to stay patient and attentive to the rider's comfort level.

7.4. Choosing the Right Horses

The horses used in therapeutic riding programs should be sound, patient, good-natured, and capable of adapting to the riders' needs. They may come from various backgrounds, but all need to undergo specific training to work in therapeutic riding. A temperament test is often useful to evaluate potential therapy horses. Care of these wonderful animals isn't a small task, either: from maintaining their health to ensuring they remain physically and mentally stimulated, horses need plenty of attention.

7.5. Training Horses

Equine training for therapeutic riding should focus on desensitization to unusual movements or objects, as well as accepting different rider positions. The horse should be able to work calmly at all riding gaits, and adapt to different situations. A variety of exercises can be included in the training process, such as leading, lunging, longlining, and eventually riding with weight bags before introducing the rider.

7.6. Volunteer Management

Volunteers often play a critical role in the running of a therapeutic riding program. Not only do they assist during sessions, but they may also help with the horses' care and facility upkeep. Ensuring they receive proper training and guidance is vital. Moreover, scheduling regular volunteer appreciation events can boost morale and retention.

7.7. Facility Requirements

The therapeutic riding program facility should be wheelchair-accessible and have a safe, clear space for mounting and dismounting the horses. It's also beneficial to have a quiet, comfortable area for riders to relax before and after their sessions, as well as for families and caregivers to wait. A clean, safe environment for the horses is equally important.

7.8. Budgeting and Funding

Start-up and maintenance costs for a therapeutic riding program can be significant. A detailed budget needs to be established that includes facility costs, horse care, salaries, utilities, and equipment. Explore opportunities for grants, sponsorships, and fundraising activities to support the program.

7.9. Program Evaluation

After the program is up and running, perform regular audits and evaluations to assess its effectiveness. Feedback from riders, families, and volunteers is invaluable. Observations from instructors and therapists are also crucial. This performance evaluation should lead to strategic improvements to better meet participants' needs.

Above all, keep the lines of communication open. An environment where everyone feels comfortable voicing their concerns or suggestions is essential for a successful therapeutic riding program.

By addressing these key areas, you can create a therapeutic riding program that provides meaningful and enjoyable experiences for participants while fostering a healing and growth-oriented environment. The process may be complex and prolonged, but the potential rewards — improved wellbeing, self-esteem, and a sense of achievement for your riders, and a sense of purpose and fulfillment for you and your team — are beyond measure.

Chapter 8. Safety Measures and Risk Management in Therapeutic Riding

Safety is paramount in therapeutic horseback riding, requiring thoughtful oversight given its dynamic nature. The harmonious blending of individuals with varying degrees of ability, horses with distinct personality traits, and often unpredictable natural environments necessitates stringent measures to manage risk.

8.1. Identifying Potential Hazards

Hazards in therapeutic horseback riding range from the handling and behavior of horses, rider's health condition and abilities, quality and suitability of equipment, environmental conditions, to the competence and training of staff and volunteers. A regular, systematic inspection should be carried out using a checklist detailing every possible risk area.

1. Equine Behavior: Horses, even the well-trained therapeutic ones, remain animals with unpredictable behaviors. An inspection should involve understanding the horses' health, temperament, and suitability for individual riders.

2. Rider's Health and Abilities: Some riders might have health conditions that could affect their balance, coordination, or control during riding. It's essential to have a thorough understanding of each client's unique needs.

3. Equipment: Tack must fit properly and be checked continually for signs of wear and tear. Poorly-fitted or worn equipment can lead to injuries.

4. Environmental Conditions: The riding area, both indoors and

outdoors, should be inspected for safety before every session. Pay attention to ground conditions, secure fencing, and no protruding objects.

5. Staff and Volunteers: Those assisting in lessons need to be sufficiently trained to manage emergencies. They should communicate effectively with riders and understand horse behaviors.

8.2. Risk Assessment

Risk in therapeutic riding is an interplay between the likelihood of an incident and its potential impact. Risk assessment involves assessing each identified hazard, determining the severity, the likelihood of occurrence, and implementing measures to control these risks. Strategies may range from eliminating the hazard entirely to reducing the hazard or controlling its impact.

8.3. Analyzing Incident Data

Analyzing past incident data is crucial for risk management. Frequent evaluation of such reports can shed light on trends, indicating areas needing more attention. This retrospective view can provide insights leading to preventive measures and improved safety protocols.

8.4. Developing An Emergency Response Plan

An essential part of risk management is having an Emergency Response Plan (ERP). The ERP should encompass provisions for various emergencies - from falls and injuries to intense weather conditions and equine emergencies. Everyone involved should be familiar with this plan and trained accordingly.

1. Incident Management: The ERP should detail the required steps to ensure all incidents are managed swiftly and efficiently, minimizing the potential for harm.

2. Medical Assistance: The plan should detail the protocol for immediate medical response and evacuation, if necessary.

3. Weather-Related Emergencies: For weather-related emergencies, the ERP should contain protocols for identifying and responding to potential weather hazards.

4. Equine Emergencies: The ERP must address sudden horse health issues or unpredictable behavior, detailing procedures to ensure both human and equine safety.

8.5. Training Staff and Volunteers

The competency of staff directly correlates to participant safety. Therefore, regular training on safety protocols is a necessity.

1. Basic Training: All staff members should be well-versed in basic safety measures such as correctly fitting helmets and other protective aids, proper mounting and dismounting techniques, emergency dismount, and fall recovery.

2. Emergency Procedures: A thorough understanding and ability to execute all the emergency procedures detailed in the ERP is paramount.

8.6. Implementing Safety Measures for Riders

The safety of the riders is central in all aspects of therapeutic riding. Implementing measures to guarantee their safety involves proper preparation before riding, during riding, and after the ride.

1. Pre-ride Preparations: This includes a physical and mental health

check, use of suitable and correctly fitted safety gear, and a brief about what to do in case of an unexpected event.

2. During the Ride: The rider, depending on their abilities, should have assistance at hand. Also, the right pacing and measured progression of sessions are essential.

3. Post-Ride: After riding, it's crucial for participants to decompress, absorb their experiences, and discuss any concerns.

8.7. Conculsion

To conclude, maintaining safety in therapeutic riding requires careful consideration, strategic planning, and continuous vigilance. From identifying potential hazards to developing an Emergency Response Plan, everyone involved - staff, volunteers, and riders - play a critical role. Through these articulated safety measures, the healing journey of therapeutic riding can indeed be an enriching, empowering, yet safe experience.

Now that you understand the necessity of safety measures and risk management in therapeutic horseback riding, the subsequent sections will delve into the nuances of rider assessment and specific riding techniques, providing insight into navigating this extraordinary journey.

Chapter 9. Suitable Activities and Techniques for Different Abilities

Therapeutic horseback riding offers an exceptional platform for people of all ability levels to benefit physically, emotionally, and psychologically. Rooted in the understanding of each participant's unique capabilities, the tailored activities and techniques involved can facilitate the achievement of specific therapeutic goals set by therapists and instructors.

9.1. The Role of the Horse

The key element in all these activities is the horse. The horse's movement gives beneficial neuromuscular and sensory input, which simulates the human gait and can be translated to improved functional ability off the horse. Also, horses, as sentient beings, offer emotional connection and motivation to riders.

9.2. Therapeutic Riding Activities by Ability Level

Let's delve into suitable activities and techniques for different abilities, considering cognitive, physical, and emotional aspects.

9.2.1. Cognitive Abilities

For participants with cognitive challenges, incorporating activities that stimulate brain functioning into riding sessions can be beneficial. By coupling the movements of riding with these activities, cognitive skills like memory, attention, and problem-solving can be improved.

- *Sequencing*: Encourage riders to remember a series of commands or cues in order. This could involve following a particular route within the riding arena or executing a series of different movements on the spot.

- *Colour or Shape Sorting*: Using coloured rings or foam shapes, ask the riders to sort or identify items according to their colour or shape while seated on the horse. This not only improves cognitive skills but also helps develop fine motor abilities.

- *Storytelling*: Incorporate story-telling into the riding session. Ask the rider to narrate an ongoing story, pausing at intervals for them to continue the narrative.

9.2.2. Physical Abilities

Therapeutic riding sessions can also be tailored for those with physical disabilities. Here are a few suggestions:

- *Balance Games*: Games that require core stability and balance can be useful. Examples of such activities might involve reaching for a ring or passing a ball while maintaining a seated position on the horse.

- *Obstacle Course*: An obstacle course can be a fun and engaging way to improve spatial awareness, motor planning, and balance. For instance, weaving between cones or going under arches requires careful planning and body adjustments.

- *Mirror Riding*: This activity involves the rider copying the movements or patterns demonstrated by the instructor either on a horse or on the ground.

9.2.3. Emotional Abilities

For individuals facing emotional challenges, therapeutic riding can offer a unique platform for building trust, confidence, and emotional control:

- *Horse Care*: As part of the therapeutic riding session, participants can be involved in grooming or feeding the horse. This provides a way to foster empathy, responsibility, and emotional connection.

- *Practicing Mindfulness*: Incorporating mindfulness activities, like deep breathing or body scans, can offer a grounding experience.

- *Creative Expression*: Encourage the riders to express their feelings or thoughts by drawing or writing about their experiences with the horse or session, which can serve as an outlet for emotions.

9.3. Adapting Techniques for Specific Disabilities

While planning therapeutic riding activities, it's crucial to adapt techniques for specific disabilities. Underneath are broad guidelines for a couple of specific conditions.

9.3.1. Autism Spectrum Disorder (ASD)

Participants with ASD might demonstrate a wide range of abilities, requiring thoughtful adjustment in riding sessions:

- *Predictability*: Keep activities consistent to create a predictable setting, as students with ASD often find comfort in routine.

- *Visual Supports*: Use visual cues to indicate the session's flow, making it easier for the individual to understand and follow instructions.

- *Sensory Activities*: Include sensory-rich activities, such as riding over different textures, which might offer a soothing experience for some individuals.

9.3.2. Cerebral Palsy

When working with riders with Cerebral Palsy, the focus is often on improving muscle control, balance, and coordination. Recommended activities include:

- *Core Strengthening*: Include balance activities, such as yoga poses on horseback, to strengthen the core muscles.

- *Multisensory Stimulation*: Use techniques that engage the rider's different senses, like the attachment of various textures around the reins that the rider can touch while riding.

Remember that each individual is unique. All activities should be customized to meet each rider's needs and therapeutic objectives, ensuring safety, enjoyment, and effective therapy.

Chapter 10. Building Trust and Bonding: The Secret to Successful Therapy

When it comes to therapeutic horseback riding, one cannot overstate the significance of trust and bonding. This relationship between the therapy participant and their equine partner forms the backbone of successful therapy. Herein, we delve deep into the process of fostering this crucial bond, it's multifaceted importance in therapy, the nuances of equine behavior, and the different methods to strengthen this extraordinary relationship.

10.1. Understanding the Basics

Understanding trust and bonding begins with an appreciation of why these aspects are foundational to the therapeutic process. Firstly, therapeutic horseback riding involves not just physical interaction, but emotional and cognitive engagement too. Thus, the formation of a safe, trusting relationship between the therapy participant and the horse becomes a prerequisite to effective therapy.

Trust and bonding ensure the rider feels secure, capable, and connected. When a therapy participant feels these positive emotions, they become progressively receptive to therapy, facilitating breakthroughs in emotional wellbeing, physical strength, and cognitive abilities.

As for the horse, trust-building makes them obedient, calm, and responsive to the rider's commands, further reinforcing the rider's confidence and control. Therefore, the concept of trust extends beyond mere companionship. It is a powerful adjunctive tool that can significantly fuel therapeutic progress.

10.2. The Nuances of Equine Behavior

To build trust and bonding with a horse, one must first understand equine behavior. Horses are herd animals and instinctively establish a pecking order. They value a calm, decisive leader who provides direction and safety. Horses also have an acute sense of intuition. They can detect human emotions and respond accordingly, sometimes even mirroring those emotions. Understanding these attributes is key to fostering a fortifying and healthy bonding.

Horses communicate non-verbally through body language. Every wag, whinny, or shuffle is a form of communication. Learning to interpret these signs paves the way to understanding the horse's mindset, thus providing valuable information to build a strong trust bond.

10.3. Committing to a Patient Approach

Trust-building with a horse is a process that requires patience. Just as it is with human relationships, it takes time for a horse to trust a new person. The pace at which horses develop trust varies from one individual to another. Hence, the therapy participant, along with their instructor or caregivers, is advised to remain patient and consistently positive in their approach.

10.4. Methods to Foster Trust and Bonding

Several methods systematically promote trust and bonding between the therapy participant and the horse, engaging at both physical and emotional levels.

Spending Quiet Time Together: Beginning with non-demanding, quiet time allows both the rider and horse to acclimate to each other's presence.

Grooming: This activity has a two-fold purpose: It allows the therapy participant to connect with the horse, while also fulfilling an essential part of the horse's care routine.

Groundwork: This includes leading the horse, lunging, turning, and halting. Such exercises give the therapy participant an opportunity to play a leadership role, thus establishing their position.

Learning Voice Commands: Teaching the therapy participant to effectively use voice commands improves communication with the horse, enabling better control and navigation.

Rewarding Good Behavior: Positive reinforcement like petting or giving a treat for good behavior encourages trust.

10.5. Cultivating Emotional Awareness

Educating the therapy participant about the empathetic qualities of horses is vital. Being aware that horses can sense and mirror human emotions encourages the participant to manage their feelings around the horse effectively. This also paves the way for emotional bonding and understanding.

10.6. Safety Measures During Trust-building

Safe interaction is the cornerstone of a healthy trust-building process. Therapy participants should be coached on safety measures like appropriate body language, maintaining safe distances, and understanding the horse's personal space. Instructors should always supervise these activities until they're confident of the participant's ability to interact safely with the horse.

In conclusion, the journey of trust-building in therapeutic horseback riding is as rewarding as it is essential. Its depth extends beyond the superficial understanding of trust, cascading into emotional understanding, deep bonding, and empowerment of the therapy participant. It's a crucial step towards effectuating optimal therapeutic progress, destined to yield a profound, lasting impact on the individual's life.

Chapter 11. Evaluating Progress and Success: The Path Forward

One of the paramount facets in the implementation of a therapeutic horseback riding program is the evaluation of progress and success. Documenting and reviewing progress not only reinforce trust in the program by generating tangible evidence of gains but also provide valuable insights for refining intervention techniques and strategies.

11.1. Define Success Parameters

In therapeutic horseback riding, success may revolve around various dimensions, including physical, cognitive, emotional, and social improvement. A well-defined and systematic approach to measure success includes the following aspects:

1. Long-term goals: These are broad objectives that the participant intends to accomplish through the program, such as enhancing their overall wellbeing, augmenting social interaction, or attaining a particular physical milestone.

2. Short-term goals: These are stepping-stones towards achieving the long-term goals, comprising specific attainable targets set in a defined time span.

3. Evaluation methods: Depending on the set goals, various methods can be adopted for evaluation, including standardized tests, direct observation, participant self-reports, caregiver or therapist reports, and recording relevant physical markers (e.g., muscle strength, flexibility, etc.).

11.2. Documenting Progress

On-going documentation using standardized templates can assist in correctly capturing the progress in therapeutic horseback riding. Here are a few pointers to consider:

1. Start with a baseline: A baseline should represent the participant's status before beginning the therapy. It provides the initial reference point against which all future comparisons can be made.

2. Regular updates: Implement regular updates to document the participant's progress towards achieving the short-term goals. Consider including quotes from instructors, therapists, or caregivers that give nuances about the participant's improvements.

3. Milestones tracking: Documenting the milestones, whether big or small, can act as an excellent morale booster for participants and a practical resource to appraise effectiveness of the program.

4. Review and revise: Regularly reassess the goals and upcoming activities based on the participant's progress. Be open to revise the plan to accommodate new challenges and opportunities.

11.3. Methods of Evaluating Progress

A combination of objective and subjective evaluation methods reinforces the validity of the results.

1. Objective evaluation: This could be gauged through physical markers, performance on a certain task, or results of standardized tests.

2. Subjective evaluation: This could pertain to a participant's or caregiver's perceived changes in behaviour, mood, or overall

quality of life.

Participant self-evaluations can also give valuable insights into their perceived progress and how the program impacts their wellbeing, offering a more holistic view of the therapy's effectiveness.

11.4. Analyzing Results

Finally, analyzing the collected data is vital to understand the efficacy of the therapeutic horseback riding program. Regular analysis can inform you of whether the program is on the right track or needs any adjustments.

1. Positive trends: Look out for gradual improvements in the results over the weeks and months. For instance, improved muscle strength or cognition, increased interaction, or improved emotional wellbeing.

2. Unanticipated results: These are unexpected outcomes that may surface during therapy, such as novel skills developed or personal discoveries made. Unanticipated results should be noted, appreciated, and integrated where feasible.

3. Adjustments to the program: Based on the analyzed data, make necessary adjustments to the program to accommodate faster progress or work on the identified challenges.

11.5. Sharing the Success

Once the progress and success have been evaluated, sharing these results with relevant stakeholders is critical. Regular updates can also serve to reinforce the therapeutic relationship, build trust, and keep the participant and their households engaged and invested in the process. Celebrating small wins and progress markers can significantly foster motivation in participants and create a positive environment for growth and healing.

Therapeutic horseback riding defies a rigid, 'one-size-fits-all' approach. It's a process that is continually shaped by the participant's evolving needs and experiences, underpinned by a robust system of documenting and evaluating progress. It's about meshing the equestrian world with a resilience-focused approach to therapy, and this chapter interprets what this courageous ride might look like in terms of evaluating and celebrating the progress and success.

www.ingramcontent.com/pod-product-compliance
Lightning Source LLC
Chambersburg PA
CBHW062310290526
45794CB00006B/2748